Guidelines for
Scientific Integrity:
A Handbook for Research

Acknowledgements

A number of individuals contributed to the development of the Third Edition of the Scientific Integrity Guidelines. We acknowledge the assistance of the following individuals who served as writers, without which this update would not have been possible.

- Helen W. Lach, PhD, RN, FGSA, FAAN, Saint Louis University (Editor)
- Kimberly Arcoleo, PhD, MPH, University of Rochester
- Claire B. Draucker, PhD, RN, APRN, FAAN, Indiana University- Purdue University Indianapolis
- Karen H. Morin, PhD, RN, ANEF, FAAN, University of Wisconsin-Milwaukee
- Ann Garwick, PhD, RN, LMFT, LP, FAAN, University of Minnesota
- Deborah Loman, PhD, RN, APRN, CPNP, Saint Louis University
- Thomas E. Stenvig, PhD, RN, MPH, NEA-BC, South Dakota State University
- Rebecca Luebbert, PhD, RN Southern Illinois University, Edwardsville
- Amy Funk, PhD, RN-BC, Illinois Wesleyan University, MNRS Emerging Scholars Network

Thanks to the following for their thoughtful review and suggestions:

- Janet Sullivan-Wilson, PhD, RN, University of Oklahoma
- Ann M. Berger, PhD, APRN-CS, AOCNS, FAAN, University of Nebraska Medical Center
- Stephanie Solomon Cargill, PhD, Saint Louis University Center for Healthcare Ethics
- Sarah Oerther, MSN, MEd, RN, Saint Louis University, MNRS Emerging Scholars Network
- Daniel L'Ecuyer, Formatting Consultant
- Pamela Richards, Editorial Consultant

Guidelines for Scientific Integrity:

A Handbook for Research

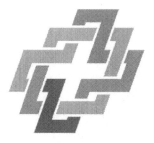

Midwest Nursing Research Society
Third Edition

ISBN-13:978-1979961820

ISBN-10: 1979961824

Published by the Midwest Nursing Research Society

2018

Table of Contents

Introduction

The first edition of this handbook on scientific integrity was published in 1997 by the Midwest Nursing Research Society (MNRS). From the preface of that edition, the authors noted "increasing confusion and uncertainty regarding issues of scientific integrity such as authorship, ownership of data, student's rights and others" (MNRS, 2002, p. ii). The authors may not have anticipated the significant interest this topic would generate over the ensuing years among parties from all sectors of the research enterprise: from students to scientists to research funders to journal editors to government oversight committees. They would be surprised by the significant research misconduct that would be identified among scientists from across disciplines. A growing body of research and literature has developed since the last edition to address the broad range of subjects related to scientific integrity.

Drawing from the second edition of the guidelines published by MNRS (2002), we maintain the objectives for this work: "a) guide research practice, b) assist in the training of young investigators, c) promote accountability in the conduct of science and serve the interests of the society, and d) stimulate dialogue, debate, and continued refinement about these and related issues" (p. v). In this new version, we build on the work of the prior authors, providing updated information, issues, and references for the current researcher. These guidelines introduce a variety of issues, and we hope students and researchers will build on what they learn here to develop a solid understanding of principles and strategies to maintain scientific integrity in their research practices.

Individual Research Practices

Integrity is defined as "honesty" and "adherence to moral and ethical principles" (Dictionary.com, 2017). For the nurse researcher, this definition applies to the practice of research. As the most trusted health professionals (ANA, 2015a), it is imperative that nurse researchers maintain scientific integrity, promote transparency in research, and avoid misconduct as key research responsibilities. Education, mentoring, policies, procedures, and federal oversight all work together to support positive research practices. In this handbook we introduce the key topics in scientific integrity and provide resources for learning more about this important topic. The goal is to support nurse researchers in their important endeavors, which we draw from the Midwest Nursing Research Society (MNRS) vision, *to improve the health of all people* (MNRS, 2016).

In this booklet, we address research broadly, although some content is only relevant to research with human subjects. Because much research conducted by nurses involves people, human subjects' issues are woven throughout the contents. Responsible conduct of research is critical whether it involves human subjects, laboratory samples, animals, or synthesis of prior literature. Nurse researchers should be familiar with all aspects of scientific integrity, and uphold standards of good practice in all their research endeavors.

Ethical Responsibilities

Scientists are guided by shared values and principles. These are respect for the integrity of knowledge, collegiality, honesty, trust, objectivity, and openness. These values are relevant to each phase of the research process. The state of knowledge and development of disciplines and subspecialties within them determine the research processes employed by scientists. Disciplines, through their social organizations, shape research practices and identify standards of conduct.

Institutional and societal environments within which research is conducted further influence these practices and standards. In addition, the individual integrity and behavior of scientists, legal requirements, and policies by governmental regulatory agencies affect research practices in a variety of ways. These all combine with regulations and laws to guide scientific practice.

Scientific Integrity

One of the most important values is that of scientific integrity, defined as "justice and honesty in proposing, conducting, and reporting research, or doing it right and telling the truth about what you did" (Khanyile, Duma, Fakude, Mbombo, Daniels, & Sabone, 2006, p. 41). Thus scientific integrity is synonymous with good scientific conduct, and is "intrinsically tied with integrity principles (honesty, reliability, objectivity, impartiality-independence, open communication, duty of care and fairness)" (Fierz, Gennaro, Dierikx, Van Achterberg, Morin, & De Geest, 2014, p. 272). Shamoo and Resnick (2015, p 15) note that scientific integrity is based on "understanding and obeying the different legal, ethical, professional, and institutional rules that apply to one's conduct." Scientists need to keep scientific integrity at the forefront of all research activities, particularly given the increasing reports of scientific misconduct within the scientific community that led to a paper in the journal *Nature* entitled "Scientists Behaving Badly" (Martinson, Anderson & de Vries, 2005).

The American Nurses Association (ANA), in *The Code of Ethics for Nurses with Interpretive Statements* (2015b), Provision 7, states "All nurses must participate in the advancement of the profession through knowledge development, evaluation, dissemination, and application to practice "(p. 27). For those conducting research, this provision means that research undertaken by nurse scientists is "necessary, soundly constructed, significant, worthwhile, and that all necessary resources are available" (Fowler, 2015, p. 117). Moreover, scientists must have a clear understanding of the ethical responsibilities associated with research, including the need to promote and maintain scientific integrity. Nurse researchers have an obligation to mentor

2

students and serve as role models of those working with them to uphold the ANA code.

Scientific Misconduct

Research misconduct has been broadly defined as "fabrication, falsification, or plagiarism in proposing, performing, or reviewing research, or in reporting research results" (Office of Research Integrity, n.d.). Other types of misconduct include failure to follow scientific regulations, incompetence, carelessness, inadequate supervision of subordinates, dishonesty, poor work environments, and problems with authorship (Keith-Spiegel, Sieber, & Koocher, 2010). Martinson, Anderson & de Vries (2005) also list dropping data, using inadequate research designs, changing methodology in response to pressure from a funder, withholding methodological details, withholding data that does not support the researcher's work, ignoring minor human subjects' requirements, and overlooking poor interpretations of data, as problems. In addition, unethical behaviors could include violations of animal research regulations, inappropriate peer review, and mistreatment of human or material research resources (Shamoo & Resnick, 2015). Individual institutions may have their own definitions of misconduct.

Nurses conducting research are not immune to poor practices, as Fierz and colleagues (2014) reported. The most common instances of scientific misconduct include misattribution of authorship; plagiarism, and data fragmentation (Egry, Barbosa, & Cabral, 2015). Broome et al. (2010) found journal reviewers also had concerns about protection of human and animal subjects in studies they had reviewed. Cases of misconduct related to federally funded projects are reviewed by the U.S. Department of Health and Human Services (DHHS) Office of Research Integrity (ORI), and findings their investigations are posted on its web site. Examples have included nursing research. According to Steneck (2007, p 21), actions considered to be misconduct should be investigated to determine if they "represent a significant departure from accepted practices, were committed intentionally, or knowingly, or recklessly, and be proven by a preponderance of evidence."

Regardless of the definition, scientific misconduct can have a broad negative impact to the research enterprise as a whole (Macrina, 2014). The challenges to individual scientists and institutions can range from embarrassment to ineligibility for funding, to legal ramifications. Institutions and trainees may be stigmatized because of their association with the scientist. There are costs and stresses to institutions investigating potential misconduct. When situations are made public, confidence in research is compromised.

When scientific misconduct is suspected, researchers have an obligation to address it. However, approaches may be informal or formal. Sometimes an observer can misunderstand a situation that is the cause of a concern. Discussion with a trusted colleague may be helpful in considering the possible explanations for the situation as well as potential actions. Institutions have guidelines on how to report issues. The individual should carefully consider what approach to take, as well as possible risks to themselves as well as those suspected of misconduct, in deciding on a course of action (see guide by Kieth-Spiegel, Sieber, & Koocher, 2010).

Historical Roots

A number of historical examples prompted increasing regulation of research with human subjects (Karigan, 2001). Prisoners were subjected to inhumane research practices in Nazi Germany during World War II, and African Americans were followed long-term in a study of syphilis without being offered treatment when it became available. In a more recent study, a healthy volunteer died from medication provided for the research, resulting in complete suspension of research at a university. These and a number of other cases of inappropriate practices have led to guidelines and regulations on research with human subjects to prevent future problems.

Formal efforts to protect research participants began following World War II. In 1947 the Nuremburg Code of ethical principles was developed. The ethical principles guiding human subjects' protections and informed consent were published in the *Declaration of Helsinki* and are updated regularly by the World Medical Association (2016). The *Belmont Report* was written by the National Commission for the Protection of Human Subjects of Biomedical and Behavioral Research (1979). The Commission was charged with identifying ethical principles, and developing guidelines for the ethical conduct of research with human subjects.

Federal regulations with guidance on responsible conduct of research and scientific integrity are available and updated by government agencies including the National Institutes of Health (NIH), U.S. Department of Health and Human Services, the Office of Human Research Protections (OHRP), and Office of Research Integrity (ORI), among others. The DHHS *Code of Federal Regulations* (1991) provided details on implementing appropriate research practices. Several Federal departments and agencies joined HHS in adopting a uniform set of rules for the protection of human subjects, the ``Common Rule,'' identical to subpart A of 45 CFR part 46 of the DHHS regulations in 1991. Although minor revisions had occurred, no large-scale modifications were made until 2017, even though the research landscape had changed dramatically. Minor changes were scheduled to go into effect in 2018, address issues such as improving consent, and changes in IRB guidelines for multisite studies, exempt studies, and continuing review. Nurse researchers should be familiar with current rules guiding research.

Guiding Ethical Principles

The foremost ethical principles guiding human subject research are autonomy (respect for persons), beneficence, and justice (Greaney, et al., 2012). Researchers address each of these issues in research proposals and protocols. Autonomy provides that individuals have free choice in deciding to participate in research without coercion. Further, participants give informed consent, with full understanding of their options, potential risks and benefits, and their ability to withdraw at any time without penalty. This principle also supports the need to protect those who are vulnerable, or who have diminished autonomy. Some individuals may not be allowed to participate in research because of this risk. For example, some states do not allow a non-family member to consent for another person to participate in research, even if

5

they hold legal guardianship. Vulnerable populations are discussed in detail later in this handbook. Other factors related to autonomy include privacy and confidentiality. Information about individuals should be kept confidential if not anonymous, and steps should be taken to protect identifiable research information.

Beneficence calls for the scientist to act in the best interest of research participants, as well as to maximize the benefits and minimize risks or potential harms related to the research. Scientists typically think of physical harms, but psychological harms can be significant, such as emotional distress, embarrassment, discomfort when disclosing information, fear of repercussions, or stigma (Polit & Beck, 2015). No research is without some risk, even if only inconvenience, possible loss of confidentiality, or mild psychological discomfort from thinking about uncomfortable topics. Researchers should consider all potential risks and plan how they will attempt to minimize risks or manage any adverse events that occur during the research process. Risks and benefits should be fully disclosed to potential participants.

Researchers track and report adverse events that occur during research activities. These should be reported and evaluated to determine if an event is related to the research. Further, researchers conducting intervention studies should set up a data and safety monitoring board (DSMB) to routinely monitor adverse events and examine study data to identify potential safety concerns (Artinian, Froelicher & Vander Wal, 2004). Studies may be stopped if untoward effects of the research are identified. In addition, new scientific information about treatment may come to light during the study that may impact the conduct of the study or participants' decisions to participate. If so, research participants may need to be informed and re-consented based on their understanding of the new information.

Justice calls for fair application of research, as well as fair inclusion of individuals (*Belmont Report,* National Commission for the Protection of Human Subjects of Biomedical and Behavioral Research, 1979). Those who may benefit from research should be included, as well as bear any burdens or risks from the research. Populations should not be used based on convenience, such as prisoners or nursing home residents. On the other hand, vulnerable populations should not be excluded from research that might benefit them specifically. Historical exclusion of some groups, such as minorities, women, children, and older adults in research studies has resulted in limitations in knowledge of how some interventions or treatments work in these populations (Taylor, 2009; Herrera et al., 2010). Nurse researchers should consider the inclusion and exclusion criteria in studies to promote fair application of research risks and benefits.

Chapter Summary

Research is guided by ethical principles, federal regulations, and institutional policies and procedures. Falsification, fabrication, and plagiarism are the primary forms of scientific misconduct. Historical events have led to increased research regulation and oversight. Nurses conducting research are responsible for maintaining scientific integrity in all aspects of their work.

Considerations for Your Research

1. What personal characteristics are important to develop as a researcher?
2. What resources do you have to help develop these characteristics?
3. How do ethical principles apply to your area of research?
4. What approaches are suggested if you thought another researcher was doing something unethical?

References

American Nurses Association. (2015a). *Nurses rank as most honest, ethical profession for 14ᵗʰ straight year.* Retrieved from http://nursingworld.org

American Nurses Association. (2015b). *Code of Ethics for Nurses with Interpretive Statements.* Silver Springs, MD: author.

Artinian, N. T., Froelicher, E. S., & Vander Wal, J. S. (2004). Data and safety monitoring during randomized controlled trials of nursing interventions. *Nursing Research, 53*(6), 414-418. doi: 10.1097/00006199-200411000-00010

Broome, M. Dougherty, M. C., Freda, M. C., Kearney, M. H., & Baggs, J. G. (2010). Ethical concerns of reviewers: An international survey. *Nursing Ethics, 17*(6), 741-748. doi: 10.1177/0969733010379177

Integrity. (2017). In *Dictionary.com* online. Retrieved from http://www.dictionary.com/browse/integrity40-years

Egry EY, Barbosa DA, Cabral IE. (2015). The many sides of research integrity: For integrity in nursing! *Revista Brasileira de Enfermagem, 68*(3):327-9. doi.org/10.1590/0034-7167.2015680301i

Fierz, K., Gennaro, S., Dierickx, K., Van Achterberg, T., Morin, K. H., De Geest, S. (2014). Scientific misconduct: Also an issue in nursing science? *Journal of Nursing Scholarship, 46* (4), 271-280. doi: 10.1111/jnu.12082

Fowler, M. D. M. (2015). *Guide to the Code of Ethics for Nurses with Interpretive statements. Development, interpretation, and Application* (2ⁿᵈ Ed.). Silver Springs, MD: American Nurses Association.

Greaney, A., Sheehy, A., Heffernan, C., Murphy, J., Mhaolrunaigh, S. N., Heffernan, E., & Brown, G. (2011). Research ethics application: A guide for the novice researcher. *British Journal of Nursing, 21*(1), 38-43. doi: 10.12968/bjon.2012.21.1.38

Herrera, A. P., Snipes, S. A., King, D. W., Torres-Vigil, I., Goldberg, D. S., & Weinberg, A. D. (2010). Disparate inclusion of older adults in clinical trials: Priorities and opportunities for policy and practice change. *American Journal of Public Health, 100* (Suppl 1), S105-S112. doi: 10.2105/AJPH.2009.162982

Karigan, M. (2001). Ethics in clinical research: The nursing perspective. *American Journal of Nursing, 101* (9), 26-31.

Keith-Spiegel, Joan Sieber, & Gerald P. Koocher (2010). *Responding to research wrongdoing: A user-friendly guide.* Retrieved from http://www.ethicsresearch.com/freeresources/rrwresearchwrongdoing.html

Khanyile, T. D., Duma, S., Fakude, L. P., Nbombo, N., Daniels, F., & Sabone, M. S. (2006). Research integrity and misconduct: A clarification of concepts. *Curationis, 29* (1), 40-45.

Macrina, F. L. (2014). *Scientific integrity: Text and cases in responsible conduct of research* (4th Ed). Washington, DC: ASM Press.

Martinson, B. C., Anderson, M. S., & de Vries, R. (2005). Scientists behaving badly. *Nature, 435,* 737-738. doi: 10.1038/435737a

Midwest Nursing Research Society (MNRS). (2016). *Improving the quality of research for more than 40 years.* Retrieved from http://www.mnrs.org

National Commission for the Protection of Human Subjects of Biomedical and Behavioral Research. (1979). *The Belmont report: Ethical principles and guidelines for the protection of human subjects of research.* Retrieved from: http://www.hhs.gov/ohrp/humansubjects/guidance/belmont.htm

Office of Research Integrity (ORI). (n.d.). *Definition of research misconduct.* Retrieved from: http://ori.hhs.gov/definition-misconduct

http://www.mnrs.org/improving-quality-nursing-research-more-

Polit, D. f. & Beck, C. T. (2017). *Nursing Research: Generating and Assessing Evidence for Nursing Practice.* 10th Ed. Philadelphia: Wolters Kluwer.

Shamoo, A. E., & Resnik, D. B. (2015). *Responsible conduct of research.* (3rd Ed.). New York: Oxford University Press.

Steneck, N. H. (2007). *ORI Introduction to the responsible conduct of research.* Office of ResearchIntegrity (ORI). Retrieved from https://ori.hhs.gov/ori-intro

Taylor, H. A. (2009). Inclusion of women, minorities and children in clinical trials: Opinions of research ethics board administrators. *Journal of Empirical Research on Human Research Ethics: An International Journal, 4*(2), 65-73. doi: 10.1525/jer.2009.4.2.65

World Medical Association (2016). *Declaration of Helsinki on ethical principles for medical research involving human subjects.* Retrieved from http://www.wma.net/en/20activities/10ethics/10helsinki/index.html

2

Institutional Responsibilities

Academic and research institutions are increasingly held accountable for supporting scientific integrity and monitoring research conduct at their institutions. A variety of regulations address scientific integrity topics such as conflict of interest, human subjects, and animal welfare. Institutions must hold or obtain a Federal Wide Assurance and follow specific regulations when they have employees conducting research with human subjects, or obtaining grants or contracts to conduct research (Office of Human Research Protections, 2011).

Institutions are accountable to the public and to research sponsors for oversight in the generation of high quality scientific knowledge, and for good stewardship of funds.
Committed institutional leadership at the highest level is critical in promoting responsible science. The goal of such leadership is to provide education in responsible conduct of research (RCR), oversee research processes, and when misconduct occurs, to take prompt and appropriate action. Institutions should create systems that encourage and reward good scientific practices. Such systems should emphasize quality over quantity, as well as provide formal guidelines and systems that take into account the values of each of the disciplines while staying in compliance with the increasing regulations. Institutional policies should be designed to protect investigators, provide for appropriate collaborations with funders or sponsors, and individuals outside the institution.

Institutions must assure researchers and collaborators are trained on the responsible conduct of research. Standard online programs are available nationally, that are usually accepted across institutions, and NIH has requirements for face to face training as well for funded researchers and

10

trainees (NIH, 2016b). Geller, Boyce, Ford & Sugarman (2010) encourage training that focuses on the ethical underpinnings of regulations, to keep the focus on protecting participants and researchers, despite some of the burdens of regulatory compliance. Further, they suggest that institutions strive for a culture that supports reporting of problems and concerns about ethical conduct, similar to that promoted by the patient safety movement.

Institutional Review Board

Research with human subjects must be reviewed by a federally approved Institutional Review Board (IRB) in the U. S. Federal regulations guide the conduct and membership of the IRB, to include researchers and non-researchers and a member not affiliated with the primary institution to prevent undue bias (Grady, 2015). The IRB reviews the risks and benefits of studies, as well as measures to assure adequate protection of subjects, especially informed consent procedures, confidentiality, identification of risks and steps to minimize them. In addition, IRBs provide continuing review over the course of the study, typically an annual review of all studies, as well as review of any adverse events that occur.

Many IRBs consider the quality of proposed studies to protect potential subjects from any risks or burdens from participating in poorly designed studies. For example, studies need sufficient numbers of subjects to answer the research questions, but no more than necessary. The goal is to assure scientific value of studies, especially with the scarce resources for conducting research (Emmanuel, Wendler & Grady, 2007).

Studies fall into one of three categories for IRB review, based on level of risk. Specific federal criteria apply for each category. Intervention study proposals with human subjects require a review by the full IRB committee review, which are then discussed at a meeting for approval. This applies to studies that have more than minimal risk and include collection of patient identifiers, which applies to most intervention studies and biomedical research. An *exempt* study typically renders no more than minimal risk to participants and provides for protection of subject identity, avoiding the need for written consent of subjects. This type of study typically does not require a full IRB board review. An expedited study is somewhere between, usually involves identifiable health information attained through interaction or data previously collected for non-research purposes, but also has only minimal risks. Often additional materials are required for IRB submissions, such as an informed consent form, or additional confidentiality protections. The researcher provides documentation, and the IRB conducts a review and makes final determination of category and approval or disapproval of projects. Successful collaboration with the IRB can be enhanced by developing relationships with IRB staff, proactively seeking advice, following guidelines, and anticipating that the process will take time (Cartwright, Hickman, Nelson & Knafl, 2013).

Privacy of Health Information

While IRBs typically address privacy of health information, the Health Insurance Portability Accountability Act (HIPAA) adds another set of regulations institutions must help researchers manage. When personal health information is collected as part of a study with identifiers, participants must be given the institution's notice of privacy practices and their signatures obtained as proof that this was received (Wipke-Davis & Pickett, 2008). HIPAA regulations may limit researcher access to patient information. For example, researchers may not be allowed to access data about patients or names of potential subjects for recruitment in clinical settings. Instead, staff at the site may be required to provide data on patients who may be appropriate for studies, or make the approach for recruitment, then refer individuals to the researcher if patients are interested and agree to be contacted (Weierbach, Glick, Fletcher, Rowlands & Lyder, 2010). Researchers need careful planning for determining potential sample populations, recruitment of subjects, and managing follow-up contacts to maintain HIPAA compliance.

Non-academic institutions often have nursing or research committees or individuals designated to oversee and approve research conducted at their sites. A letter of support is usually needed to submit to the IRB from research sites outside the university or approving IRB institution. Researchers need to work with clinical sites or research partners to garner support and develop methodologies that will be feasible and acceptable to these sites.

Conflict of Interest

Conflict of interest (COI) is defined by the Institute of Medicine (2009, p. 6) as "circumstances that create a risk that that professional judgement or actions regarding a primary interest will be unduly influenced by a secondary interest." In research, conflicts have the potential to impact ethical conduct of research due to other interests. Informal influences can come from such sources as pressures to succeed, or attain funding or tenure. Conflicts of commitment or over-commitment of time to many projects can reduce attention to projects. External relationships or financial incentives related to a study may cause concern about monetary influence on research findings.

Increasingly, scientists have relationships with industry or are developing products with potential to provide financial gain. Almost a quarter of nursing journal reviewers reported concerns about COI in a survey by editors (Broome, Dougherty, Freda, Kearney, & Baggs, 2010). However, having a COI does not mean the researcher is doing anything wrong, but rather the potential exists for bias in the research process. Steps can be taken to identify sources of conflict and reduce the potential for influence on research.

Institutions must identify and address financial conflicts of interest among their researchers. Once identified, a process to review conflicts and identify a plan to manage the conflict is required. Options include eliminating the conflict, or developing a plan to manage the conflict and increase transparency (Lach, 2014). Management plans may include such actions as disclosing the conflict to research staff and participants, as well as in any publications. In other instances the conflicted researcher may be excluded from participating in the informed consent process. Oversight of data analysis by a non-conflicted researcher may be required. Institutions may avoid making contracts with funders or sponsors that limit or prevent investigators from accessing, analyzing or publishing data from funded studies.

Most journals today require a statement of potential conflicts from authors, which are published with the study. The goal is to increase transparency in the research process. Researchers should be aware of potential conflicts of interest, develop plans to manage any conflicts, and avoid arrangements with outside entities that impact transparency of research, such as limits on analysis or reporting of data.

Quality Improvement Research

Nurse researchers may be involved in evidence-based practice projects such as quality improvement (QI) projects, or mentoring trainees on QI projects. The question of whether these are considered "research" and require IRB review is a common question (Cacchione, 2011). Quality improvement projects may be conducted by organizations for their own internal development, while research is defined as "a systematic investigation, including research development, testing, and evaluation designed to develop or contribute to generalizable knowledge" (USDHHS, 1991). Hospital staff, faculty, as well as Clinical Nurse Leader and Doctor of Nursing Practice (DNP) students conduct these kinds of projects. If aggregate data are used, such as run charts from a unit, IRB may not be needed. When studies include individual data, with a goal to publish the findings, they may require IRB review.

Other considerations that may move QI into the research category include the following (adapted from McNett & Lawry, 2009):
- Evaluation of a drug or device, or an intervention that is not current standard of care
- Collection of protected health information
- Testing a change of practice in some patients but not others, or comparing one or more interventions among different patients
- Causing patients to potentially experience risks or burdens that are beyond standard practice (i.e. collecting information you would not normally collect, or doing something you would not normally do in delivering patient care)

Ultimately, individual IRBs will make the final decision about the need for review. Nurse researchers may submit a summary of potential projects to the IRB for help in making determinations.

Sometimes nurse researchers complete a QI project and then later decide they would like to share or publish findings that might benefit others. Submission of a retrospective study may be appropriate. The local IRB can provide guidance on steps to take in this situation. However, planning for potential publication, and obtaining approvals beforehand is preferred.

Animal Research

Nurses are increasingly conducting basic research including studies with animals to examine physiological responses to phenomena that can't practically be studied in humans. Research with animals is carefully regulated to promote humane treatment. Oversight of animal care and approval of studies is provided by an Institutional Animal Care and Use Committee (IACUC), similar to the IRB for human subject research (National Institutes of Health, 2016). Researchers should provide a strong rationale for use of animals in research, and assure that the selection of the animal and any procedures applied offer the appropriate model to answer the research question. Further, nurse scientists need training, planning, and resources in order to conduct research using animals appropriately (Holtzclaw & Hanneman, 2002).

Chapter Summary

Institutions are responsible for oversight of research processes to promote scientific integrity. All human subjects' research must be reviewed and approved is reviewed by an Institutional Review Board. Other institutional responsibilities include research involving animals, financial conflicts of interest, and managing privacy of health information. Quality improvement projects may be a form of institutional research.

Considerations for Your Research

1. What are the training requirements at your university or institution regarding responsible conduct of research?
2. Are you familiar with the resources at your university or institution related to research that address requirements and regulations?
3. What factors impact the level of IRB review needed (exempt, expedited, full review)? Are you familiar with the forms and guidelines of the IRB at your university or institution?
4. Are you aware of any conflicts of interest that might affect your research?

References

Broome, M. Dougherty, M. C., Freda, M. C., Kearney, M. H., & Baggs, J. G. (2010). Ethical concerns of reviewers: An international survey. *Nursing Ethics*, 17(6), 741-748. doi: 10.1177/0969733010379177

Cacchione, P. Z. (2011). When is institutional review board approval necessary for quality improvement projects? *Clinical Nursing Research*, 20(1), 3-6. doi: 10.1177/1054773810395692

Cartwright, J. C., Hickman, S.E., Nelson, C. A., & Knafl, K. A. (2013). Investigators' successful strategies for working with institutional review boards. *Research in Nursing & Health*, 36, 478-486. doi: 10.1002/nur.21553

Emmanuel, E. J., Wendler, D., & Grady, C. (2007). What makes clinical research ethical? *Journal of the American Medical Association*, 283 (20), 2701-2711. doi: 10.1001/jama.283.20.2701

Grady, C. (2015). Institutional review boards: Purpose and challenges. *Chest*, 148(5), 1148-1155. doi: 10.1378/chest.15-0706

Geller, G., Boyee, A., Ford, D., & Sugarman, J. (2010). Beyond compliance: The role of institutional culture in promoting research integrity. *Academic Medicine*, 85, 1296-1302. doi: 10.1097/ACM.0b013e3181e5f0e5

Holtzclaw, B. J., & Hanneman, S. K. (2002). Use of non-human biobehavioral models in critical care nursing research. *Critical Care Nursing Quarterly, 24(4), 30-40.*

Institute of Medicine (IOM). (2009). *Conflict of Interest in Medical Research, Education, and Practice.* Washington, DC: The National Academies Press.

Lach, H.W. (2014). Financial conflicts of interest in research: Recognition and management. *Nursing Research, 63, 228-232.* doi: 10.1097/NNR.0000000000000016

McNett, M., & Lawry, K. (2009). Research and quality improvement activities: When is institutional review board needed? *Journal of Neuroscience Nursing, 41, 344-347.*

National Institutes of Health (NIH). (2016). *What investigators need to know about research with animals.* Retrieved from https://nih.gove/grants/policy/air/policy.htm

National Institutes of Health (NIH). (2016b). *Responsible conduct of research training.* Retrieved from https://oir.nih.gov/sourcebook/ethical-conduct/responsible-conduct-research-training

Office for Human Research Protections (OHRP). (2011). *Federal wide assurance for the protection of human subjects.* Available http://www.hhs.gov/ohrp/register-irbs-and-obtain-fwas/fwas/fwa-protection-of-human-subjecct/index.html

U. S. Department of Health and Human Services (USDHHS). (1991). Code of federal regulations, Title 45, Part 46, Protection of Human Subjects. *Federal Register, 56, 28003-28024.* Available at http://www.hhs.gov/ohrp/regulations-and-policy/regulations/45-cfr-46/

Weierbach, f. M., Glick, D. F., Fletcher, K., Rowlands, A., Lyder, C. H. (2010). Nursing research and participant recruitment: Organizational challenges and strategies. *Journal of Nursing Administration, 40(1), 43-48.* doi: 10.1097/NNA.0b013e3181c97afb

Wipke-Tevis, D. D. & Pickett, M.A. (2008). Impact of Health Insurance Portability Act on Participant Recruitment and Retention. *Western Journal of Nursing Research, 30(1), 39-53.* doi: 10.1177/0193945907302666

3

Protection of Human Subjects

The researchers' primary responsibility is to assure that participants in studies are treated ethically and protected from undue risks. Certain populations are vulnerable to coercion and exploitation in research. Potential risks and vulnerabilities should be identified and plans for minimizing these threats incorporated into study protocols.

Informed Consent

The most important mechanism for protecting research participants is through the informed consent process. Informed consent assumes the following: disclosure of the risks and benefits and activities of the study by the researcher, and then understanding, voluntariness, and capacity of the participant to give consent. The researcher is obligated to assure that clear explanations are given about the study. Researchers must assess understanding of research protocols and assure that participants have capacity to consent. Finally, participation must be voluntary without coercion. For example, incentives can be provided to compensate participants for their efforts, but should not be so excessive as to be coercive or provide undue inducement, thus compromising voluntariness.

Consent forms are written with the subject population in mind, addressing such issues as educational level and health literacy. The elements of consent must be included in forms (DHHS, 2016), and should be clear, whether a signed consent form is required or researchers are able to use a recruitment statement or verbal consent (e. g. for conduct telephone screening). When obtaining informed consent, multiple communication modes are suggested to improve understanding, (Cohn & Larson, 2007), such as a combination of written information, verbal explanations, use of other media, as well as assessment of participant understanding.

The teach-back method can be used to confirm participant understanding of the purpose of the study and what they are being asked to do (Agency for Healthcare Research and Quality, 2012).

Researchers must disclose what they know about risks and benefits of studies, but even with clear explanations, potential participants may have misperceptions. Therapeutic misconception can be a significant threat to informed consent if study participants inappropriately confuse research with clinical care (Horng & Grady, 2003). While there may be potential benefits to subjects when they participate in studies, research goals are different from clinical care and not typically individualized to the participant. Clinical trials of medical interventions are particularly subject to this confusion. Therapeutic misestimation is when participants are not clear on the purpose, or the probability of risks or benefits, expecting better outcomes than may be likely. The researcher should assure that study participants make a decision to participate with appropriate expectations. A mild form of misconception is therapeutic optimism, where participants hope for positive outcomes from research participation. A positive attitude is not itself problematic, and may be a good thing, unless it contributes to more significant misunderstanding (Horng & Grady, 2003). Researchers should provide adequate disclosure regarding study participation and assess participants' understanding of the potential benefits of what they are consenting to do.

Vulnerability in Research

Vulnerability in research can be considered along two dimensions based on participant capacities (Goldfarb, 2006): These include "capability" (i.e., able to understand information about the study and make an informed decision about participation) and "autonomy" (i.e., able to make a decision without influence or coercion)." The *Code of Federal Regulations* (DHHS, 1991) has added additional protections for populations they identify as "vulnerable." These include but are not limited to, prisoners; pregnant women; human fetuses and neonates; and children. Special federal regulations and protections are required for research with these specific groups. Other groups, such as those who are decisionally-impaired individuals, employees, economically disadvantaged individuals and those with sensitive health problems may be considered to be vulnerable populations by individuals IRBs. Unequal power relationships may constitute vulnerability. Special precautions should be taken, for example, to ensure autonomy for groups such as students, marginalized populations, individuals with poor health literacy, and those dependent on others for care. Collection of sensitive information and certain types of studies also may place individuals at risk.

Researchers should be cognizant of the particular circumstances that render potential subjects vulnerable. Individuals who are imprisoned or institutionalized, for example, may fear retaliation for refusal to participate in research. Those who have mental health or emotional issues may be vulnerable to psychological harms. Battered women may be at risk for retaliatory violence if their research involvement is discovered by abusive partners or ex-partners. Persons living with AIDS or other stigmatized illnesses may be jeopardized if information they reveal about their health status became public. While these groups may need special protections, some researchers argue against over-labeling of vulnerable groups that may reinforce stigma, and hinder research that may address their important health needs (DuBois et al., 2012). Research may help address problems of vulnerable groups. Researchers should determine the risks of a study and particular vulnerabilities of potential subject populations and then provide appropriate protections without overprotecting or stereotyping vulnerable groups.

When conducting research with vulnerable populations, nurse researchers are especially attuned to maintaining privacy and confidentiality, securing fully informed consent, avoiding coercion in recruitment and retention of subjects, and enhancing the psychological and physical safety of participants. Language and health literacy issues should always be considered, particularly in immigrant or marginalized populations. Vulnerable groups should not be overused as research participants because of their
availability, nor should they be routinely excluded from research that would be advantageous to them. Justice

demands fair distribution of both the benefits and burdens of research.

Practices that enhance socially responsible research with vulnerable groups include making visible the historical, economic, and social contexts of the lives of participants; involving participants or affected community members in research planning; using multiple methodologies to discover and present participant perspectives that might be silenced by traditional approaches, and being keenly aware of how research findings might be used to advance progressive or repressive social policies (Fine, Weis, Weseen, & Wong, 2000). The following sections introduce key issues among some common vulnerable populations that research scientists may encounter.

Vulnerable Populations

Prisoners. Prisoners are vulnerable because of limited autonomy and potential for coercion (Miracle, 2010). However, research may be relevant to their circumstances and benefit this population. Special guidelines are provided to assure protections. The recruitment and selection of prisoners for research should be performed in a random manner of those who meet criteria. Any incentives to prisoners for research participation should not be viewed as coercive or impair decision-making (OHRP, 2003).

Pregnant Women, Fetuses and Neonates. Research involving these populations is also subject to special considerations in order to provide adequate protections (DHHS, 1991). IRBs carefully consider potential risks, including what is known about risks from animal studies or studies in other populations along with benefits of the research. Both the pregnant woman and fetus need to be considered (Beattie & VondenBosch, 2007). Consent of fathers may be needed for pregnant women to participate in research; non-pregnant women are not considered vulnerable, even if they could become pregnant during a research study (Miracle, 2010). Conditions under which research with fetuses and neonates may be conducted are specified in federal regulations and state regulations may apply.

21

Children. Minors and children are considered vulnerable because they "are persons who have not attained the legal age for consent to treatments or procedures involved in the research" by the OHRP (2016). The OHRP further provides guidelines on approval of projects for IRBs based on risks and benefits. Four types of research are permitted, including studies that pose no more than minimal risk. Research may have more than minimal risk, if there is potential benefit to the participant, if there is adequate societal benefit, or if the study provides an opportunity to learn more about important problems affecting children. Determining the exact level of risk can be challenging. For example, children with chronic illnesses such as cancer may have very different life experiences than healthy children that must be considered (Beattie and VandenBosch, 2007).

Both written informed consent from parents/guardian and assent from children 7 years and older should be obtained based on the developmental maturity of the child. Research participation should be described to children in a developmentally appropriate manner and include the potential benefits, risks and required study activities (NAPNAP, 2014). Adolescents may be allowed to consent to studies on specific topics or circumstances where the state has determined that these youth are mature minors or emancipated (English, Bass, Boyle & Eshragh, 2010). Nurse researchers must consider age and development in design of studies and informed consent procedures.

Patients. Researchers who are healthcare providers may experience a conflict between the best interest of the patient and the best interest of science when involving their own patients in research. Providers can potentially have undue influence on patients when asking them to participate in research, and voluntariness may be affected if patients feel obliged to participate for their provider (Campbell-Crofts, Field, Fetherstonhaugh, 2013). Further, when a provider recruits a patient, there is increased risk of therapeutic misconception. Clinicians must clarify their dual roles, and it may be more appropriate to have another member of the research team recruit participants to promote voluntariness among participants (Steinke, 2004), and clarify the purposes of research studies. Issues related to specific vulnerable patient populations are discussed separately.

Researchers may learn information in the course of research requiring intervention, even if participants are not their own patients. For example, untreated physical or mental health issues or serious risks may be uncovered; for example: suicidal ideation. Because of the depth of sharing in qualitative studies, this possibility is enhanced (Eide & Kahn, 2008). Researchers should consider potential issues that may be uncovered, and spell out methods for addressing situations that may arise in study protocols, such as how to refer participants for assistance if needed. Another approach is to provide all study participants with information about resources for potential problems that may come up during a study (e. g. depression, intimate partner violence).

Decisional Impairment. There is much debate on how to determine whether an individual is competent to understand the many implications of research participation in order to provide a truly voluntary informed consent. Assessment of decisional capacity is best determined according to four psycho-legal standards: the ability to state or express a choice, the ability to comprehend relevant information, the ability to appreciate the situation and its likely consequences, and the ability to manipulate information rationally (Appelbaum & Grisso, 1988). Researchers have explored ways to assess consent capacity.

The first standard, to state a choice, refers to the individual's ability to communicate the choice. While this choice may be expressed orally, nonverbally, or in writing, it is important to note that *failure to object* is not equivalent to voluntary agreement. The ability to comprehend relevant information, the second standard, refers to the participant's ability to comprehend information regarding the nature of the research, including any foreseeable risks and benefits.

The third psycho-legal standard is the ability to appreciate the situation at hand. This standard requires that the person not only understand the procedures and foreseeable risks and benefits (as in the second standard), but must also then acknowledge how these issues relate to his or her own personal situation and individual circumstances. The fourth and final criterion is the ability to manipulate information rationally. This standard is the most stringent of the four and requires that participant has the ability to weigh the risks and benefits of the various options and then arrive at a "reasonable" decision as to whether participation in the research would be in his or her best interest (Fisher, 2003).

A person who is able to demonstrate these four standards should be considered capable of acting as self-governing agents and make independent decisions regarding research participation. To deny individuals who demonstrate these capacities that right is to deny them of the fundamental principle of autonomy and self-determinism. It is important that decisional capacity be assessed not only when obtaining consent prior to study participation, but throughout the duration of the study. This is especially important if the participant has a condition whereby cognition may be affected over time. Diminished capacity to give informed consent in certain populations can be permanent, fluctuating or progressive (Beattie and VandenBosch, 2007).

When presenting study information to a prospective research participant, the study presentation must be clear and concise. The researcher should use simple lay language that is easily understood by the participant. While some participants may ask frequent questions to clarify an issue, others may opt not to ask questions for fear that they may appear resistant or not intelligent. Therefore, in the event that a person is not asking questions, it is important for the researcher to ask questions that evaluate the participant's understanding of the presented materials. Participants should be provided with copies of consent documents and also contact information of the researchers. Lines of communication between the researcher and participant should be open through the duration of the study in the event that issues arise (Luebbert & Perez, 2016).

Mental Health. While laws declare that people with mental illness have the right to provide consent to participate in research, little is understood about the extent to which mental illness may hinder a person's capability to make decisions that will be in his or her best interest. Overall, two issues are raised. First is the concern that impaired decisional capacity of some individuals may result in refusal of needed treatments they would likely have obtained had they possessed the capacity to comprehend the benefits of the offered research. The second concern is that impaired decisional capacity may result in acceptance of unnecessary treatments that may have otherwise been refused. As a result, there tends to be two beliefs by professionals. Some assert that mental illness invariably impairs decisional capacity to the extent that a participant is no longer competent to make independent decisions regarding research participation. On the contrary, others assert that those with mental illness are just as capable as those without such illnesses to provide an independent consent (Grisso & Appelbaum, 1995).

To minimize potential bias toward those with mental illness, it is imperative for the researcher to assess decisional capacity of participants on an individual basis as with other illnesses. Failure to do so would stigmatize individuals with mental illness, denying their basic human right to research participation, and also potentially limit much needed research of psychiatric conditions (Luebbert, Tait, Chibnall, & DeShields, 2010).

Older adults. Older research participants may be vulnerable due to medical conditions that are common with age, impacting autonomy and informed consent. However, healthy older adults without such issues may not be any more vulnerable than other adults (Walsh, 2009). Medical conditions may impair sensory systems (vision, hearing) and ability to understand information. Other conditions impact decisional capacity such as Alzheimer's disease causing progressive loss of memory and judgement. In these cases, consent of a legal representative should be obtained, but in addition, assent of the impaired person to participate should be obtained at the time of research activities. Assessment of cognitive status may be needed when conducting research in older adults, and specific protections may be needed when targeting cognitively impaired populations (Beattie, 2009).

Residents of long-term care facilities may be vulnerable because they are often frail with multiple chronic diseases, and may be dependent on others for care, or may not feel comfortable refusing to participate in studies. Engagement of staff from institutions and communities when developing and implementing studies can improve ethical conduct of research in long term care settings (Lingler, Jablonski, Bourbonniere, & Kolinowski, 2010). Protocols may need to address how potential safety information will be addressed if uncovered during research, such as elder abuse or depression and suicidality as health providers may be mandatory reporters. Nurse researchers should develop protocols that support ethical engagement of older participants, including use of larger fonts, reading consent forms, assuring appropriate environments (lighting, noise), use of cognitive assessments, and follow-up procedures.

Acute, Critical, or Terminal Illness. Individuals with acute or critical illness may not have decisional capacity for providing informed consent, and burdens of research participation have to be considered. This can affect patients as well as family members who may be recruited to studies. They may be worried about an ill family member or under stress themselves. Even after consent, the current condition of the participant and demands of the study must be assessed at each point of contact including severity of illness and symptoms such as pain (Tait, 2009), and cognitive state. Those with terminal illness may be especially vulnerable, and unlikely to benefit personally from research (Polit & Beck, 2017). Studies should be designed to minimize impact on patients' health care and comfort, and assure autonomy in informed consent.

Employees. Special consideration may need to be given when recruiting nurses or others who are employees of an institution as research participants (Resnik, 2016). A statement in the consent form/letter should state that participation will in no way affect employment at the institution. If nurse administrators or managers are involved as investigators, special safeguards are needed against real or perceived coercion of subordinates being asked to participate. Identities of respondents should be protected. Institutions may request that direct line managers not have access to data with employee identification. If employees are unionized, there may be additional requirements. The institutional review board or human resource personnel may assist researchers in this area to plan appropriate procedures.

Students. Educational research is valuable, and student engagement in research is enticing as a strategy to mentor, foster intellectual growth, and stimulate interest in research among students. But students represent a potentially vulnerable group for nurse researchers. Respect for persons mandates the capacity for self-determination free from controlling interference, and the ability to give informed consent must be assured in research involving students (Greaney et al., 2011).

If nurse scientists in a faculty role are responsible for instruction or advising of students who are potential research subjects, an inherently unequal power relationship exists with potential for coercion of students who may fear adverse consequences of refusal to participate. For this reason, students should not be asked directly to consider participation but given the opportunity to respond with assent via neutral means of communication (Schwenzer, 2008). Another option is to defer recruitment to people who are not faculty for potential research subjects, and if possible, keep identities from being disclosed. Incentives should be appropriate for the time and effort involved. There should be no possibility of negative influence on assignment or course outcomes for those who choose not to participate (Aycock & Currie, 2013). For example, if extra credit is provided for research participation, a non-participation option should be provided. If data collected primarily for student assignments and pedagogical reasons is used for secondary purposes such as research external to measuring student achievement, potential conflict of interest should be avoided and the research should be empirically justified, outlining potential student benefits of such analysis while not compromising learning (Kirkwood, 2012).

Vulnerability Related to Research Design/Approach

Sensitive Information. The risks of loss of confidentiality are increased in studies where sensitive information is addressed (e.g., illegal behaviors; sexual attitudes, preferences or practices, HIV/AIDS, violence or abuse, suicide). Qualitative methods may be best to explore such topics (Elmir, Schmied, Jackson, & Wilkes, 2011). In qualitative studies, sensitive information may be revealed as participants become comfortable with researchers. Extra protections may be required in study procedures to protect confidentiality.

Nurse scientists need to be aware of laws that may require reporting of information uncovered during research (i.e. child abuse or elder abuse) and address these in informed consent procedures as well as study protocols. In addition, research data may be subject to subpoena for legal reasons. A possibility to prevent this is to obtain a Certificate of Confidentiality from the National Institutes of Health (2017). This prevents the researcher from being required to disclose information in any civil, criminal, administrative, legislative, or other proceeding, whether at the federal, state, or local level (NIH, date). Typically, Certificates are in effect from the date of issuance through the expiration date of the study and this protection is permanent for the coverage period. The study does not have to be federally funded to obtain a Certificate of Confidentiality.

Genetics Research. Genomic research is an expanding area and individual privacy and protection of protected health information is essential. Family and even community members may need to be involved if shared genetic information could be revealed. This concern is relevant for some racial or ethnic groups and people with rare diseases. A lapse may result in discrimination or stigma towards the individual, family or community. A discussion of the participant's desire to receive genetic findings should occur in advance (NIH, 2015). Data sharing of genetic data is encouraged by NIH but there should be consent by the individual for secondary data analysis and researchers should abide by the most current NIH guidelines (NIH, n.d.).

Big Data. The increase in large databases that can and are being used in research may provide new opportunities for improving health. Nurse researchers are increasingly involved with this type of research (Westra, 2016). However, the potential risk and ethical issues are just lately being explored, and standards for use may not exist. There are potential issues with privacy, and who and where information can be shared, and IRBs will examine risks and benefits of such studies. Recently, calls for oversight and attention to vulnerable populations have been reported (Donia, 2015). Increased training of scientists and students in these methods is needed to increase nursing contributions in this area.

Internet Research. Increasingly studies are conducted via survey or using data collected with online methods. These methodologies are appealing due to the ease of obtaining data and ability to reach populations easily. However, these methods have potential ethical problems, particularly related to autonomy and confidentiality. Recruitment should still allow for full informed consent. Often surveys include a recruitment statement in lieu of written consent, and screening questions to assure that appropriate participants respond to the survey. Completion of surveys implies consent or response items confirming consent can be included before completing the survey (Longo, 2010). While participants may feel comfortable refusing to participate in online research, once they begin a survey, forced choice questions may reduce autonomy of participants in a way that could limit their participation.

Confidentiality can be an issue due to risks of hacking. While secure systems should always be used, alerting online study participants of potential breaches in confidentiality may be required related to privacy of information (Williams, 2012). Researchers sometimes collect data from online chatrooms or other public or social media sources. Steps should be taken to protect those participants and follow the guidelines of the online site. Watson, Jones, & Burns (2007) suggest a framework for ethical planning of studies using data from such sites.

Other ethical issues may arise in Internet research. Threats to data collection include potential inability to identify who is providing information. For example, duplicate surveys may be submitted or individuals may submit information for others (i.e., spouse fills out questionnaire). Beyond usual ethical issues with research in children, legal issues can arise as data cannot be collected from children under 18 (Williams, 2012), who may inadvertently participate. When collecting sensitive information, or if studies have psychological risks, researchers need to provide help for follow up or resources for participants if needed, such as contact information of the researcher or helpful web sites (Longo, 2010). Further, populations may be excluded from online studies as access to the internet may still be a disparity. The Association of Internet Research (2012) offers guidelines for ethical decision making for researchers conducting research using the internet. Nurse researchers should consider ethical implications in designing online studies.

International Research. Ethical principles for research apply to international research as well as studies completed in the United States, to prevent vulnerabilities. All research proposals should be evaluated by an institutional, regional, or national research ethics committee within the country of the study. The population under study should benefit from the knowledge gained from the research. The purpose of the research should be described to potential participants as well as the potential risks and benefits as part of the informed consent process (World Health Organization, 2011).

With the expansion of global health research and the increased attention paid to research ethics and training initiatives, there has been a shift in the focus on ethical concerns related to reducing potential for exploitation. Effective international research collaborations and partnerships are needed that attend to cultural, community, and context differences as well as power and resource imbalances (Harrowing, Mill, Spiers, Kulig, & Kipp, 2010; LeBaron, Iribarren, Perri, & Beck, 2015; Meslin, Were & Akuku, 2013; Millum, Grady, Keusch & Sina, 2013). It is noteworthy that the International Centre for Nursing Ethics formed the Working Group for the Study of Ethical Issues in

Nursing Research (Olsen et al., 2003) and published guiding principles of (a) respect for community, and (b) contextual caring to the standard Western principles of (c) respect for persons, (d) beneficence, and (e) justice for the ethical conduct of international research.

In conducting international research in low and middle-income countries (LMICs), investigators need to consider a variety of factors. These include (a) the balance between risks and benefits, (b) provision for the care and compensation of participants if injuries occur, (c) assuring informed consent and participant understanding of any risks involved, (d) fair treatment of participants regardless of personal characteristics, (e) equitable distribution of burdens and benefits of research, and (f) potential availability of treatments, should the treatment under investigation prove effective (National Bioethics Advisory Commission, 2001). Researchers have been focusing on improving the quality of informed consent in LMIC countries through different modes of administration and addressing health literacy levels (Dawson & Kass, 2005; Madava, Pace, Campbell, Emanuel, & Grady, 2012; Montalvo & Larson, 2014; Tamariz, Palacio, Robert & Marcus, 2013).

Some have argued that many of the ethical concerns in international health research are similar to those in the United States. However, differences in context, setting, culture, and other norms in developing countries shed a different light on issues pertaining to protection of human subjects. In addition, unlike developed countries, sometimes governmental structures and legal protections may be absent for assurance of protections. Oversight of research may be lacking. This creates a situation that requires vigilance on the part of investigators.

A number of organizations collaborate to provide guidance on the ethical conduct of international research: the Council for the International Organizations of Medical Science (CIOMS), the World Health Organization (WHO), and the International Centre for Nursing Ethics (CIOMS, 2002). Substantive guidelines related to ethical principles and procedural or operational requirements are provided by these organizations. They recommend ethical review of international studies by an independent group to assure compliance with ethical principles, as well as governmental regulations. In most instances, these regulations include both those required in the United States, as well as the country where the research is being conducted. The OHRP has additional information about standards and ethical issues in international research (OHRP, n. d.).

Chapter Summary

Researchers are obligated to identify and disclose potential risks and benefits to obtain voluntary informed consent from study participants. A variety of circumstances can increase the vulnerability of subjects, such as being patients, students, or having conditions that alter decision making that may impact voluntariness or risks of research. Certain approaches to research may also increase vulnerability such as genetic research. Researchers need to identify factors that affect participant vulnerability and design studies that protect participants as much as possible.

Considerations for Your Research

1. What are the risks besides loss of confidentiality that you need to disclose to obtain informed consent?
2. What is the potential for therapeutic misconception or therapeutic misestimation in your study?
3. What factors may make your research participants vulnerable?
4. What protections can you build into your study design to maximize the protection of vulnerable subjects?

References

Agency for Healthcare Research and Quality. (2012). *The AHRQ informed consent and authorization toolkit for minimal risk research.* Retrieved from https://www.ahrq.gov/funding/policies/informedconsent/index.html

Appelbaum, P. S., & Grisso, T. (1988). Assessing patients' capacities to consent to treatment. *New England Journal of Medicine, 319*(25), 1635-1638. doi: 10.1056/NEJM198812223192504

Association of Internet Research. (2012). *Ethical decision-making and internet research: Recommendations from the AOIR Ethics Working Committee* (Version 2.). Retrieved from http://aoir.org/ethics/

Aycock, D. & Currie, E. (2013). Minimizing risks for nursing students recruited for health and educational research. *Nurse Educator, 38*, 56-60. doi: 10.1097/NNE.0b013e3182829c3a

Beattie, E. R. & VandenBosch, T. M. (2007). The concept of vulnerability and the protection of human subjects in research. *Research and Theory for Nursing Practice: An International Journal, 21*(3), 156-172.

Beattie, E. (2009). Research participation of individuals with dementia: Decisional capacity, informed consent, and considerations for nurse investigators. *Research in Gerontological Nursing, 2*(2), 94-102. doi: 10.3928/19404921-20090401-01

Campbell-Crofts, S. Field, J., & Fetherstone, D. (2013). Ethical considerations for nurses undertaking research with a potentially vulnerable population with chronic kidney disease. *Renal Society of Australia Journal, 9*(2), 74-79.

Cohn, E. & Larson, E. (2007). Improving participant comprehension in the informed consent process. *Journal of Nursing Scholarship, 39*(3), 273-280. doi: 10.1111/j.1547-5069.2007.00180.x

Council for the International Organizations of Medical Science (CIOMS). (2002). *International ethical guidelines for biomedical research in human subjects.* Retrieved from http://cioms.ch/publications/layout_guide2002.pdf

Dawson, L., & Kass, N. E. (2005). Views of US researchers about informed consent in international collaborative research. *Social Science & Medicine, 61*(6), 1211-1222. doi: 10.1016/j.socscimed.2005.02.004

Department of Health and Human Services. (2016). *Informed consent checklist.* Retrieved from http://www.hhs.gov/ohrp/regulations-and-policy/guidance/checklists/

Donia, J. (2015). *It's time for a big data code of ethics.* Huffington Post. Retrieved from http://www.huffingtonpost.ca/josepph-donia-ethics_b_6941.html

DuBois, J.M., Beskow, L., Campbell, J., Dugosh, K., Festinger, D., Hartz, S., James, R., & Lidz, C. (2012). Restoring balance: A consensus statement on the protection of vulnerable research participants. *American Journal of Public Health, 102,* 2220-2225. doi:10.2105AJPH.2012.300757

Eide, P., & Khan, D. (2008). Ethical issues in the qualitative researcher-participant relationship. *Nursing Ethics, 15*(2), 199-207. doi: 10.1177/0969733007086018

Elmir, R., Schmied, V. & Jackson, D. & Wilkes, L._(2011). Interviewing people about potentially sensitive topics. *Nurse Researcher.* 19(1), 12-16. doi: 10.7748/nr2011.10.19.1.12.c8766

English, A., Bass, L., Boyle, A. D., & Eshragh, F. (2010). *State minor consent laws: A summary.* (3rd ed.). Chapel Hill, NC: Center for Adolescent Health & the Law. Available at http://www.freelists.org/archives/hilac/02-2014/pdftRo8tw89mb.pdf

Fine, M. Weis, L., Weseen, S. & Wong, L. (2000). For Whom? Qualitative research, representations and social responsibilities. In N. K. Denizen, & Y. S. Lincoln (Eds,), *Handbook of qualitative research* (2nd Ed) (pp. 107-131). Thousand Oaks: SAGE.

Fisher, C. B. (2003). Goodness-of-fit ethic for informed consent to research involving adults with mental retardation and developmental abilities. *Mental Retardation and Developmental Disabilities Research Reviews, 9*(2), 27-31. doi: 10.1002/mrdd.10052

Goldfarb, N. M. (2006). The two dimensions of subject vulnerability. *Journal of Clinical Research Best Practices, 2*(8), 1-3. doi: 10.1097/ACM.0b013e3181e5f0e5

Greaney, A., Sheehy, A., Heffernan, C., Murphy, J., Mhaolrunaigh, S. N., Heffernan, E., & Brown, G. (2011). Research ethics application: A guide for the novice researcher. *British Journal of Nursing,* 21(1), 38-43. doi: 10.12968/bjon.2012.21.1.38

Grisso, T., Appelbaum, P. S., Mulvey, E. P., & Fletcher, K. (1995). The MacArthur treatment competence study, II: Measures of abilities related to competence to consent to treatment. *Law & Human Behavior, 19,* 127-148.

Harrowing, J. N., Mill, J., Spiers, J, Kulig, J., & Kipp, W. (2010). Culture, context and community: Ethical considerations for global nursing research. *International Nursing Review,* 57(1), 70-77. doi: 10.1111/j.1466-7657.2009.00766.x

Horng, S., & Grady, C. (2003). Misunderstanding in clinical research: Distinguishing therapeutic misconception, therapeutic misestimation, & therapeutic optimism. *IRB: Ethics and Human Research,* 25(1), 11-16.

Kirkwood, K. W. (2012). The professor really wants me to do my homework: Conflicts of interest in educational research. *American Journal of Bioethics, 12*(4), 47-48.

LeBaron, V. T., Iribarren, S. J., Perri, S. & Beck, S. L. (2015). A practical field guide to conducting nursing research in low- and middle-income countries. *Nursing Outlook, 63*(4), 462-473. doi: 10.1016/j.outlook.2015.02.003

Lingler, J. H., Jablonski, R. A., Bourbonniere, M., & Kolinowski, A. (2009). Informed consent to research in long-term care settings. *Research in Gerontological Nursing, 2*(3), 153-161.doi: 10.3928/19404921-20090428-03

Longo, J. (2010). Being connected: The use of the internet for nursing research. *Southern Online Journal of Nursing Research, 10(4),* 222-233. Retrieved from http://ojni.org/issues/?p=1708

Luebbert, R.A., Tait, R.C., Chibnall, J.T., & Deshields, T. (2008). IRB member judgments of decisional capacity, coercion and risk in medical and psychiatric studies. *Journal of Empirical Research on Human Research Ethics, 3*(1), 15-24. doi: 10.1525/jer.2008.3.1.15

Luebbert, R.A. & Perez, A. (2016). Barriers to clinical research participation among African Americans. *Journal of Transcultural Nursing, 27*(5), 456-463. doi: 10.1177/1043659615575578

Mandava, A., Pace, C., Campbell, B., Emanuel, E. & Grady, C. (2012). The quality of informed consent: Mapping the landscape. A review of empirical data from developing and developed countries. *Journal of Medical Ethics, 38*(6), 356-365. doi: 10.1136/medethics-2011-100178

Meslin, E. Were, E. & Ayuku, D. (2013). Taking stock of the ethical foundations of international health research: Pragmatic lessons from the IU-MOI Academic Research Ethics Partnership. *Journal of General Internal Medicine, 28* (Suppl 3P, S639-S645. doi: 10.1007/s11606-013-2456-7

Millum, J., Grady, C., Keusch, G., & Sina, B. (2013). Introduction: The Fogarty International Research Ethics Education and Curriculum Development Program in historical context. *Journal of Empirical Research on Human Research Ethics, 8*(5), 3-16. doi: 10.1525/jer.2013.8.5.3

Miracle, V. (2010). Vulnerable populations in research. *Dimensions of Critical Care Nursing, 29*(5), 242-245. doi: 10.4103/2229-3485.106389

Montalvo, W. & Larson E. (2014). Participant comprehension of research for which they volunteer: A systematic review. *Journal of Nursing Scholarship, 46*(6), 423-431. doi: 10.1111/jnu.12097

National Association of Pediatric Nurse Practitioners (NAPNAP). (2014). *NAPNAP position statement on protection of children involved in research studies.* Retrieved from https://www.napnap.org/sites/default/files/userfiles/about/NAPNAP_PS_Children_Involved_in_Research-Studies_2014.pdf

National Bioethics Advisory Commission. (2001). Ethical and policy issues in international research: Clinical trials in developing countries. *Volume 1. Report Recommendations of the National Advisory Commission.* Retrieved from: https://bioethicsarchive.georgetown.edu/nbac/clinical/Vol_1.pdf

National Human Genome Research Institute. (2014). *Intellectual property and genomics.* http://www.genome.gov/19016590

National Institutes of Health (NIH). (n.d.). *Genomic data sharing.* Retrieved from http://grants.nih.gov/grants/policy/coc/background.htm

National Institutes of Health (NIH). (2015). National Human Genome Research Institute. *Human subjects research in genomics.* Retrieved from http://www.genome.gov/27561533

National Institutes of Health (NIH). (2017). Certificates of confidentiality: Background information. Retrieved from https://humansubjects.nih.gov/coc/background

Office for Human Research Protections (OHRP). (n.d.). *International.* Available at http://www.hhs.gov/ohrp/international/index.html

Office for Human Research Protections (OHRP). (2003). *Guidance on involvement of prisoners in research 2003.* Available at http://www.hhs.gov/ohrp/regulations-and-policy/guidance/prisoner-research-ohrp-guidance-2003/

Office for Human Research Protections (OHRP). (2016). *Special protections for children as research subjects.* Retrieved from http://www.hhs.gov/ohrp/regulations-and-policy/guidance/special-protections-for-children/index.html

Olsen, D. P., and the Working Group for the Study of Ethical Issues in International Nursing Research. (2003). Ethical considerations in international nursing research: A report from the International Centre for Nursing Ethics. *Nursing Ethics, 10*(2), 122-137.

Polit, D. f. & Beck, C. T. (2017). *Nursing Research: Generating and Assessing Evidence for Nursing Practice.* 10th Ed. Philadelphia: Wolters Kluwer.

Resnik, D. B. (2016). Employees as research participants: Ethical and policy issues. *IRB: Ethics and Human Research,*38 (4), 11-16.

Schwenzer, K. J. (2008). Protecting vulnerable subjects in clinical research: Children, pregnant women, prisoners, and employees. *Respiratory Care, 53,* 1342-1349.

Steinke, E.E. (2004). Research ethics, informed consent, and participant recruitment. *Clinical Nurse Specialist,* 18(2), 88-97.

Tait, R. (2009). Vulnerability in clinical research with patients in pain: A risk analysis. *Journal of Law and Medical Ethics, 37*(1), 59-72. doi: 10.1111/j.1748-720X.2009.00351.x

Tamariz, L., Palacio, A., Robert, M., & Marcus, E. (2013). Improving the informed consent process for research subjects with low health literacy: A systematic review. *Journal of General Internal Medicine, 28*(1), 121-126. doi: 10.1007/s11606-012-2133-2

U. S. Department of Health and Human Services (USDHHS). (1991). Code of federal regulations, Title 45, Part 46, Protection of Human Subjects. *Federal Register, 56,* 28003-28024. Available at http://www.hhs.gov/ohrp/regulations-and-policy/regulations/45-cfr-46/

U. S. Department of Health and Human Services (USDHHS). (2011). *Human Subjects Research Protections: Enhancing Protections for Research Subjects and Reducing Burden, Delay, and Ambiguity for Investigators.* Available at httpx://sss.gpo.gov/fdsys/pkd.FR-2011-07-26/html/2011-18792.htm

Walsh, S.E. (2009). Conducting research with the elderly: Ethical concerns for a vulnerable population. *Southern Online Journal of Nursing Research, 9*(4). Retrieved from http://www.resourcenter.net/images/snrs/files/sojnr_articles2/Vol09Num04Art03.html

Watson, M., Jones, D. & Burns, L (2007). Internet research and informed consent: An ethical model for using archived e-mails. *International Journal of Therapy and Rehabilitation, 14(9),* 396-403. doi: 10.12968/ijtr.2007.14.9.24580

Westra, B., Clancy, T. R., Sensmeier, J., Warren, J. J., Weaver C., & Delaney, C. W. (2015). Nursing knowledge: Big data science implications for nurse leaders. *Nursing Administration Quarterly, 39* (4), 304-310. doi: Retrieved from 10.1097/NAQ.0000000000000130

Williams, S. G. (2012). The ethics of internet research. *Online Journal of Nursing Informatics, 16*(2). Available at http://ojni.org/issues/?p=1708

Working Group for the Study of Ethical Issues in International Nursing Research. (2003). Ethical considerations in international nursing research: A report from the International Centre for Nursing Ethics. *Nursing Ethics, 10*(2), 122-137. doi: 10.1191/0969733003ne587oa

World Health Organization (WHO). (2011). *Standards and operational guidance for ethics review of health-related research with human participants.* WHO: Geneva, Switzerland. Retrieved from http://apps.who.int/iris/bitstream/10665/44783/1/9789241502948_eng.pdf?ua=1&ua=1

4

Study and Data Management Issues

Nurse scientists are responsible for appropriate management of research studies as principal investigator (PI) as well as the work of others involved with a study. This includes all of the operational details to assure the study is in compliance with regulations as well as standards for good research practices. The increase in team science means projects may be increasingly complex and challenging to manage. Clear detailed protocols should describe all research activities, who will conduct them and when and how team members will be trained. Ideally procedures are pilot tested to identify potential mishaps that can occur.

Regular team meetings and oversight assures adherence to protocols, appropriate documentation, and timely reporting of any issues. Oversight and routine monitoring of data collection, data entry and interactions with participants should be ongoing. Errors or nonadherence such as use of a wrong consent form, or failure to notify the IRB of minor protocol changes or adverse events, can occur without appropriate planning or by overextended investigators (Neely et al., 2016). Additional challenges may arise when staff members from clinical sites are involved, including staff turnover, fidelity to research procedures and communications (Mentes & Tripp-Reimer, 2002). The PI should assure ethical practices in informed consent, following study protocols, maintaining confidentiality, managing data, monitoring adverse events, analyzing, and disseminating findings as core responsibilities.

Data Management

Data management is an important component of study management in six areas according to the ORI: data selection, data collection, data analysis, data handling, data reporting

38

and publishing, as well as data ownership (ORI, n.d.). Data can take many forms, particularly when considering qualitative studies (Lin, 2009) which may include various kinds of recordings, notes, transcripts or photographs, in addition to questionnaires or survey data. Key principles involve the integrity and stewardship of the data, confidentiality, and collaboration.

Principles for data management support good research practices including the following points.

- The research team decides on data to be collected and procedures appropriate for each project (i.e. methods for collecting and recording information), and assures that team members are trained on these protocols.
- Data from clinical sources are collected following protocols, with only approved identifiers and are based on approved methods.
- Collected data are converted to a retrievable format (i.e. copied and uploaded or scanned to computer files) for archiving. Hard copies of data are carefully stored, accessible only to the study team.
- Online data are password protected and encrypted; identifiers and data are ideally stored on separate servers. Check with your information technology experts on approved ways to share or send data (i.e. encrypted e-mail, shared drives).
- Data entry, de-identification, cleaning, and analysis follow standard practices (i.e. double entry of data).
- Codebooks or dictionaries, and tracking materials should be developed and maintained so that data values are clear, and decisions about data manipulation documented.
- Data are retained with the PI as custodian, according to institution and sponsor requirements, usually 5- 7 years.
- Data are shared with team members as determined in the protocol; all are responsible for confidentiality of data. Data may potentially be shared with individuals at the PI's institution, IRB, funders, or sponsors as required, which should be disclosed in consent forms.
- Investigators are encouraged to provide other researchers, including graduate students, with access to their data for the purposes of secondary analysis, replication, or meta-analysis. Data must be de-identified. Funded studies may have data sharing requirements.

- The PI may not have ownership of data, which is subject to requirements of institutions or funders. Clinical agencies may maintain ownership of patient data, or have restrictions about use. Often grants are provided to institutions rather than individuals. The institution then owns the data rather than the PI. If the investigator moves to a new institution or university, institutional and HIPAA regulations may impact what and how research data can be transferred or moved.

Collaboration

Research collaborations have become expected and more complex with the focus on team science. Teams commonly include researchers from a variety of disciplines and institutions, including partnerships between students/faculty and academia/business. International research collaborations will continue to grow in relation to globalization (Horner & Minifie, 2011). More diverse and geographically dispersed research teams impact ethical issues surrounding authorship, peer review, conflict of interest, data, human subjects' protection, and accountability. A need exists for centralized practices and educational materials that keep up with the changing nature of collaborative science (Horner & Minifie, 2011; Ulrich et al., 2015).

Team training is needed to improve team knowledge of others and shared methods, communication and assertiveness skills, and attitudes that promote team cohesion (National Research Council, 2015). Formalizing the roles of all team members, as well as expectations and strategies for managing changes in team members or team member absences is helpful (Happell, 2010). Authorship in particular is an issue that must be negotiated among team members, which is addressed in detail in chapter 5.

Communication skills are the key to successful research leadership and effective collaboration. Open dialogue among team members is needed at all phases of research to establish trust among team members, define responsibilities, gain an understanding of individual perceptions, and effectively deal with conflict and misunderstanding within the team (Horner & Minifie, 2011; Ulrich et al., 2015). Global teams need to ensure a culturally competent research environment. Strong and ethical leadership by senior researchers guides responsible practice and ethical behavior, in addition to protecting students and junior faculty that are vulnerable to exploitation (Ulrich, et al., 2015). As previously noted, the principle investigator is responsible for oversight of collaborations and ethical practices.

Mentorship

Knowledgeable, engaged, and trusted mentors will develop quality nursing research leaders among students and beginning investigators. Not only can effective mentors provide education and guidance with research development and implementation, but also assist mentees in adapting to organizational culture and facilitating career development. Models of mentorship are broadening from senior nurses in the mentee's home setting to distance mentoring across institutions and even countries.

New researchers will learn ethical and responsible practices from their mentors both formally through instruction and informally through observation and collaboration. In fact, the mentoring relationship may be more influential in problematic ethical behavior than formal training (Anderson et al., 2007). Mentors also have a serious ethical responsibility to trainees, who have reported such vulnerabilities as not being given proper authorship or acknowledgement, overwork, poor advice, intimidation and favoritism (Horner & Minifie, 2011, p. S332; Ulrich et al., 2015). The increase in distance education and mentoring increases the need for communication and planned connections (Lach, Hertz, Pomeroy, Resnick & Buckwalter, 2013). Mentees have a responsibility as well, to communicate their goals and learning needs, and problems encountered in their research experiences to seek guidance from research mentors.

The following suggestions were adapted from the ORI (2016) to promote research integrity among students or trainees:
1. Take time to develop relationships with mentees, discuss their work and provide advice on problems.

2. Examine mentee's raw data to check for any intentional or unintentional errors.
3. Discuss both mentor and mentee expectations, to identify roles and responsibilities.
4. Identify trainees' individual strengths and weaknesses and provide needed guidance.
5. Know institutional resources and share with trainees: discuss training available and how to report ethical issues, misconduct, or other issues.

Chapter Summary

Principal investigators are responsible for managing all aspects of a research study and activities of team members. Collaborations are increasing in research; team members need training and oversight. A significant activity is managing study data, making sure to follow regulations. New researchers need strong mentoring to develop research skills and ethical practices.

Considerations for Your Research

1. Who owns the data from your study? What should you do if you should plan to move to a different institution?
2. What skills do you need to develop to manage research studies?
3. Who can provide mentoring to help you develop strong research management skills?

References

Anderson, M., Horn, A., Risbey, K., Ronning, E., De Vries, R., & Martinson, B. (2007). What do mentoring and training in the responsible conduct of research have to do with scientists' misbehavior? Findings from a national survey of NIH-funded scientists. *Academic Medicine, 82*(9), 853-860. doi: 10.1097/ACMob013e31812f764c

Happell, B. (2010). Protecting the rights of individuals in collaborative research. *Researcher, 17*(2), 34-43. doi: 10.7748/nr2010.01.17.2.34.c7460

Horner, J., & Minifie, F. D. (2011). Research ethics II: mentoring, collaboration, peer review, and data management and ownership. *Journal of Speech, Language & Hearing Research, 54*(1), S330-45. doi: 10.1044/1092-4388(2010/09-0264)

Lach, H. W., Hertz, J. E., Pomeroy, S. H., Resnick, B., & Buckwalter, K. C. (2013). The Challenges and benefits of distance mentoring. *Journal of Professional Nursing, 29*(1), 39-48. doi: 10.1016/j.profnurs.2012.04.007

Lin, L. C. (2009). Data management and security in qualitative research. *Dimensions of Critical Care Nursing, 28*(3), 132-137. doi: 10.1097/DCC.0b013e31819aeff6

Mentes, J. C. & Tripp-Reimer, T. (2002). Barriers and facilitators in nursing home intervention research. *Western Journal of Nursing Research, 24*(), 918-936. doi: 10.1177/019394502237702

National Research Council. (2015). *Enhancing the Effectiveness of Team Science*. Committee on the Science of Team Science, N.J. Cooke and M.L.Hilton, (Eds.). Washington, DC: The National Academies Press.

Neely, J. G., Paniello, R. C., Graboyes, E. M., Sharon, J. d., Grindler, D. J., & Nusssenbaum, B. (2014). Practical guide to understanding clinical research compliance. *Otolaryngology-Head and Neck-Surgery*. 150(5), 716-721. doi: 10.1177/0194599814524895

Office of Research Integrity (ORI). (n.d). *Overview of data management*. Retrieved from: https://ori.hhs.gov/education/products/n_illinois_u/datamanagement/dmotopic.html

Office of Research Integrity (ORI). (2016). *New infographic: 5 ways supervisors can promote research integrity*. Retrieved from http://ori.hhs.gov/blog/new-infographic-5-ways-supervisors-can-promote-research-integrity

Ulrich, C. M., Wallen, G. R., Naixue, C., Chittams, J., Sweet, M., & Plemmons, D. (2015). Establishing good collaborative research practices in the responsible conduct of research in nursing science. *Nursing Outlook, 63*(2), 171-180. doi: 10.1016/j.outlook.2014.10.007

5

Ethical Publication Practices

Dissemination of high quality research in retrievable formats is critical to the development of a strong nursing knowledge base (Smith, Haigh, & Jackson, 2014). Further, high standards of scientific integrity related to publication practices provide a strong foundation for the advancement of nursing science. Ethical issues in publication practices, including accurate allocation of authorship credit and upholding ethical scientific standards in publishing research findings, have received increased public and professional scrutiny (Smith, Haigh, & Jackson, 2014).

As a result of increasing concerns regarding integrity in research dissemination, several international initiatives have provided guidance for those involved in publication practices, including authors, editors, and reviewers. The Committee on Publication Ethics (2015) for example, is an international organization that provides a forum for editors and publishers to discuss publication ethics and provides a variety of other resources such as a Code of Conduct that outlines best practices in publication ethics, a variety of flowcharts to guide responses to suspected misconduct, an e-Learning Course, discussion documents, and a monthly newsletter.

Allocation of Authorship Credit

Because authorship of academic publications establishes public accountability for scientific work, is essential to the sustainability of research programs, and has implications for professional recognition and advancement, the identification and ordering of authors on publication bylines warrants careful consideration (Al-Herz, Haider, Al-Bahhar, & Sadeq, 2013; Smith, Haigh, & Jackson, 2014).

In order to promote ethical publication practices related to authorship allocation, the follow guidelines are suggested:

1. Authors should only include those who made a substantial intellectual contribution to the published work. Honorary or gift authorship is the addition of persons to an author list to show courtesy to colleagues or to enhance the legitimacy of the work. Ghost authorship is the failure to list individuals who have made important contributions to writing the work such as professional authors(Al-Herz, Haider, Al-Bahhar, & Sadeq, 2013; Grandfield, 2014; Kennedy, Barnsteiner, & Daly, 2014; Strange, 2008).

2. Researchers should use established guidelines to determine authorship credit. The most widely adopted recommendations for authorship allocation were developed by The International Committee of Medical Journal Editors (ICMJE). The ICMJE (2015) recommend that authorship be based on the following four criteria: "(1) Substantial contributions to the conception or design of the work; or the acquisition, analysis, or interpretation of data for the work; AND (2) Drafting the work or revising it critically for important intellectual content; AND (3) Final approval of the version to be published; AND (4) Agreement to be accountable for all aspects of the work in ensuring that questions related to the accuracy or integrity of any part of the work are appropriately investigated and resolved (p. 2)." Individuals who meet less than four criteria should be considered contributors and listed in the acknowledgments with their contributions specified.

3. The ranking or ordering of authors in a byline is determined by relative contributions. The first author has made the major contribution to the work, while the corresponding author is responsible for communicating with the publication team and the readership. The role of last or senior author can be conferred on the person who has directed or overseen the work and should not be conferred solely due to position in the institution, such as department chair, or preeminent standing in the field of study (Strange, 2008). In addition, middle authors should be ordered according to their relative contributions to the work.

4. The conferring or ordering of authorship should be negotiated among team members including students, preferably in advance to the writing of the publication (Sommers, 2011; Welfare & Sackett, 2010). Order may be reassessed if contributions change.
5. All authors are expected to review the final version of the manuscript and take responsibility for the work.

Ethical Practices of Scientific Writing

All authors are responsible for the quality and accuracy of work presented in publications. In order to promote publication practices that promote scientific integrity, the following guidelines are suggested:

1. Nurse researchers avoid the practices of duplicate or redundant publications (i.e., the publishing of identical or highly similar articles or major components of articles in more than one journal), text recycling (i.e., the publishing of a condensed version of previously published text), salami reports (i.e., the reporting of multiple or fragmented findings from a single study), self-plagiarism (i.e., the reuse of the author's own words without appropriate citation), or plagiarism (i.e., the use of other authors' words without appropriate citation) (Graf et al., 2014; Henly, 2014; Johnson, 2006).
2. Authors present sufficient information about a study's design so that other scientists can replicate the findings, report and justify the use of procedures that deviate from the original study design, and ensure that no false or fabricated data or manipulated photographic images are included (Graf et al., 2014).
3. Authors should include statements confirming that all required legal and ethical approvals were obtained for a study (Graf et al., 2014).
4. Authors should provide information regarding the registration of clinical trials if applicable (Graf et al., 2014).
5. Authors should disclose any funding or support for studies and any conflicts of interest related to the work.

Editors' Responsibilities

Journal editors have an important role in maintaining the integrity of science through maintaining high standards of publication ethics. COPE (2015) has published Best Practices for Journal Editors. Editors' responsibilities related to scientific integrity include:

1. Educating authors and reviewers about scientific integrity in publication practices and developing or supporting policies that reduce scientific misconduct, including processes to promote accurate authorship allocation.
2. Establishing processes to promote the thorough and accurate reporting of research results. Journals may require standardized reporting of work. Examples of publication guidelines that may be expected by journals include the Consolidated Standards of Reporting Trials (CONSORT, 2010) checklist for randomized clinical trials, the Preferred Reporting Items for Systematic reviews and Meta-analyses (PRISMA) framework (Moher et al., 2009), and the Standards for Quality Improvement Reporting Excellence (SQUIRES, 2017) guidelines.
3. Requiring authors and reviewers to disclose all relevant conflicting or competing interests.
4. Ensuring that all research published in the journal has received high quality peer review by recruiting and maintaining a diverse group of peer reviewers with expertise consistent with the journal's purpose, monitoring the performance of the peer reviewers, and providing guidance for them on matters such as providing unbiased and constructive reviews, identifying possible research misconduct in submissions, and being alert to redundant publications and plagiarism.
5. Maintaining a strong editorial board by recruiting highly-qualified board members with suitable expertise, providing clear guidance about their expected responsibilities, consulting them regularly regarding journal challenges, and providing training regarding peer review and journal management.
6. Developing procedures to ensure that commercial considerations do not affect editorial decisions.
7. Developing systems to detect plagiarized text.

8. Ensuring that authors provide evidence of ethics approvals.
9. Securely archiving published material
10. Providing authors with timely publication decisions.

Peer Reviewers' Responsibilities

Peer reviewers of scientific works submitted for publication have an important role in promoting scientific through maintaining high standards of publication ethics. COPE (2013) published Ethical Guidelines for Peer Reviewers. Peer reviewer responsibilities related to scientific integrity include:

1. Providing thorough, expert, unbiased, constructive, and timely reviews on manuscripts submitted for publication based on a fair assessment of their strengths and weaknesses.
2. Reporting all potential personal, professional, or financial conflicting or competing interests according to journal policies.
3. Maintaining confidentiality of all manuscript and review information.
4. Reporting to the editor(s) any concerns about the ethical aspects of the work, including breaches of publication ethics, such as redundancy and duplication of published works, or scientific misconduct that occurred during the research.

Retraction

Articles may be retracted if sufficient ethical problems are identified, such as major plagiarism, or the study is unethical (COPE, 2009) and may infer stigma to authors. This action can be initiated by authors or editors, but the final decision lies with the editor. Most journal databases will continue to list the paper along with a notice of retraction. Authors may identify minor errors after publication. In these cases, the editor should be notified, and corrections may be subsequently published in a future issue (Conn, 2013).

Predatory Journals

Nurse scientists should only publish in reputable journals and avoid disseminating their work in predatory journals. Predatory journals are publications that use a profit-driven author-pay publishing model, but engage in practices that lack scientific integrity and often rely on unscrupulous marketing practices to engage authors and editors (Peternelj-Taylor, 2015; Yucha, 2015). For example, predatory journals may use names of experts for their editorial boards without permission, or may not provide appropriate peer review of articles. Predatory journals are often open access, but there are many open access journals that are not considered predatory. Many disciplines publish in such journals today and pay for their publications (see copyright below for more on open access), if the journal and publisher is credible. The International Academy of Nursing Editors (INANE) has developed guidelines for evaluating the integrity of a journal, including ensuring that the editor is reputable, that the journal has a transparent and thorough process for quality control, and has sound business and publishing practices (INANE "Predatory Publishing Practices" Collaborative, 2014).

Copyright

Authors should be aware of copyright laws related to their publications. A copyright protects the written, graphic, and musical expression of ideas (Lyons, 2010) but not of the actual ideas. Examples of copyrighted material are those that are put into a tangible form, such as written material, audio or video recordings, or computer programs (Mays & Macrina, 2014). Ownership of a copyright may be held by one or more authors, the author's employer or by the publisher. These works are considered copyright-protected even without such a declaration on the manuscript or other creative work. Works that are produced by U.S. government agencies (i.e. Centers for Disease Control, Agency for Healthcare Research & Quality), or have expired copyright are copyright free and in the public domain, or available for use without permission.

For many scholarly journals, the author is required to transfer the copyright of the published article to the publisher. However, authors may negotiate to retain intellectual property rights for content or instruments that may be published, if arranged at the time of paper acceptance. Authors may do this to retain rights to a tool or questionnaire. Students may want to explore this if they want to include a published journal article in their dissertations later. Student dissertations are usually published in an online database, which may be a requirement for graduation. When students publish papers from dissertation works later in peer-reviewed journals, there is rarely a copyright issue. However, students may want to request an embargo or delayed release of their dissertations from these databases. University policies may also impact ownership of student work and should be reviewed (Kearney, 2014).

There are now numerous open access journals as noted above. Open access refers to a system of immediate on-line access to scholarly works with limited copyright restriction other than author recognition (Lyons, 2010). Scholars can download articles for free. Authors are not required to transfer copyright to an open access journal, although they give the journal exclusive rights over dissemination. Many traditional journals now offer an open access option for a fee.

With both traditional and open access journals, authors are allowed to share their published articles in a manner consistent with the signed agreement. Nurse researchers should be familiar with copyright requirements when publishing their work. They should also investigate the quality of the journal prior to manuscript submission, since some journals that have lower standards have names that are similar to well-established professional journals. These are often called predatory journals.

Intellectual Property

The term 'intellectual property' includes inventions, discoveries, technology or scientific developments, computer software, survey instruments, images, and other tangible products (World Intellectual Property Organization, n. d.). Usually, the author or developer is the 'owner' except when

50

the work-for-hire rules apply. In that instance, the employer is technically the owner. Employers, however, generally do not assert ownership unless the product has market value. Nurse researchers who conduct studies related to the development of intellectual property should review their employers' policies regarding ownership. There may be differences in copyright and ownership of work created by faculty versus staff and students.

Research data may be viewed as intellectual property and ownership should be clarified with any funding sources and affiliated institutions, as noted above. Institutions who receive grants often own data from these studies (May & Macrina, 2014). Typically, scientists must maintain data for a period of time following data collection. Most universities have policies regarding intellectual property that may impact a variety of research activities, and nurses should become familiar with these policies.

Chapter Summary

Dissemination of research findings is the final obligation of the researcher. Authors, editors, and reviewers each have a role to play in ethical publication practices. Decisions about authorship should be based on accepted guidelines. Researchers need to be aware of copyright issues and institutional policies regarding intellectual property.

Considerations for Your Research

1. Have you discussed authorship credit with any collaborators on your research?
2. What are your obligations as a journal article reviewer?
3. Have you developed instruments or materials? Have you considered if you should try to retain the copyright?
4. How do you determine appropriate journals for submitting articles?

References

Al-Herz, W., Haider, H., Al-Bahhar, M. & Sadeq, A. (2013). Honorary authorship in biomedical journals: How common is it and why does it exist? *Journal of Medical Ethics, 0,* 1-3. doi: 10.1136/medethics-2012-101311.

Committee on Publications Ethics (COPE). (2009). *Retraction guidelines.* Retrieved from http://publicationethics.org/files/retraction%20guidelines_0.pdf

Committee on Publications Ethics (COPE). (2013). *COPE Ethical Guidelines for Peer Reviewers.* Retrieved from http://publicationethics.org/files/Ethical_guidelines_for_peer_rev iewers_0.pdf

Committee on Publications Ethics (COPE). (2015). *COPE Best Practice Guidelines for Journal Editors.* Retrieved from http://publicationethics.org/files/Code_of_conduct_for_journal_ed itors_Mar11.pdf

Conn, V. S. (2013). To err is human: Managing mistakes in manuscripts. *Western Journal of Nursing Research, 35*(7), 827-828. doi: 10.1177/0193945913482547

Consolidated Standards of Reporting Trials (CONSORT). (2010). *CONSORT 2010 checklist.* Retrieved from http://www.consort-statement.org/

Graf, C., Deakin, L., Docking, M., Jones, J., Joshua, S., McKerahan, T., Ottmar, M., Stevens, A., Wates, E., & Wyatt, D. (2014). Best practice guidelines on publication ethics: A publisher's perspective, 2nd Edition. *Headache: The Journal of Head and Face Pain, 54,* 1619-1643. doi: 10.1111/head.12455

Grandfield, K. (2014). Why editors should never be "ghost" or "gift" authors. *Nursing Ethics, 21(3), 374-375.* doi.10.1177/0969733014520895

Henly, S. J. (2014). Editorial: Duplicate publications and salami reports. *Nursing Research, 63*(1), 1-2. doi:10.10.1097/NNR.0000000000000015

International Committee of Medical Journal Editors (ICMJE). (2015). *Defining the Role of Authors and Contributors.* Retrieved fromhttp://www.icmje.org/recommendations/browse/roles-and-responsibilities/defining-the-role-of-authors-and-contributors.html

International Association of Nursing Editors (INANE). (2014). Predatory publishing: What editors need to know. *Nurse Author & Editors, 23* (3), 1-5. Retrieved from http:/www.nurseauthoreditor.com/article.asp?id=216.

Johnson, C. (2006). Repetitive, duplicate, and redundant publications: A review for authors and readers. *Journal of Manipulative and Physiological Therapeutics, 29*(7), 505-509. oi:10.1016/j.jmpt.2006.07.001

Kearney, M. H. (2014). Who owns a dissertation, and why does it matter? *Research in Nursing & Health, 37,* 261-264. doi: 10.1002/nur.21611

Kennedy, M. S., Barnsteiner, J., & Daly, J. (2014). Honorary and ghost authorship in nursing publications. *Journal of Nursing Scholarship, 46*(6), 416-422. doi:10.1111/jnu.12093

Lyons, M.G. (2010). Open access is almost here: Navigating through copyright, fair use, and the TEACH Act. *Journal of Continuing Education in Nursing, 41,* 57-64. doi: 10.3928/00220124-20100126-03

Mays, T. D. & Macrina, F. L. (2014). Research data and intellectual property. In Macrina, F. L. (2014). Ed. *Scientific integrity: text and cases in responsible conduct of research* (4th Ed). Washington, DC: ASM Press.

Moher, D., Liberati, A., Tetzlaff, J., Altman, D. G., & The PRISMA Group. (2009). Preferred reporting items for systematic reviews and meta-analysis: The PRISMA statement. *Annals of Internal Medicine,* 151 (4), 264-269.

Peternelji-Taylor, C. (2015). Editorial: What authors need to know about predatory publishing. *Journal of Forensic Nursing, 11*(1), 1-3. doi. 0.1097/JFN.0000000000000064

Smith, G. D., Haigh, C., & Jackson, D. (2014). Editorial: Coping with publication ethics. *Journal of Clinical Nursing, 23,* 3293-3295. doi: 10.1111/jocn.12686

SQUIRE. (2017). SQUIRE 2.0 Guidelines. Retrieved from http://squire-statement.org/index.cfm?fuseaction=Page.ViewPage&pageId=47

Strange, K. (2008). Authorship: Why not just a toss of the coin? *American Journal of Physiology Cell Physiology, 295*(3), C567-C575. doi: 10.1152/ajpcell.00208.2008

Sommers, M. S. (2011). Negotiating journal authorship: Strategies and hazards. *Clinical Nursing Research,* 20(2), 115-119.

U.S. Copyright Office. (updated 2014). *Copyright.* Available at: http://www.copyright.gov/

Welfare, L. E., & Sackett, C. R. (2011). The authorship determination process in student- faculty collaborative research. *Journal of Counseling & Development, 89*(4), 479-487. doi: 10.1002/j.1556-6676.2011.tb02845.x

World Intellectual Property Organization (WIPO). (n.d.). *What is intellectual property?* Retrieved from http://www.wipo.int/about-ip/en/

Yucha, C. (2015). Predatory publishing: What authors, reviewers, and editors need to know. *Biological Research for Nursing, 17*(1), 5-7. doi:10.1177/1099800414563378

6

Future Developments

About sixteen years ago, the original authors of this guideline on Scientific Integrity discussed the progression of science that rings true today: "Science and scientific paradigms evolve as new and competing concepts are incorporated into existing science. Such change may come about through evolution or revolution. As with new scientific paradigms, new methods of conducting and disseminating nursing research are being developed" (MNRS, 2002, p. 17).

Today, we see new research measures, tools, and approaches implemented by nurse scientists. These new methodologies may bring with them new ethical challenges to be identified and managed. How will we protect individuals' rights to privacy? Digital data may not be secure, but can be hacked. DNA may be the ultimate personal identifier. New technological methods and artificial intelligences are increasingly available to monitor and record individual's daily lives. We look forward to discovering what new challenges will need to be addressed in the next version of this guideline! The emerging scholars of today will be writing the next versions of this guideline for future researchers.

Reference

Midwest Nursing Research Society (MNRS). (2002). *Guidelines for Scientific Integrity*. Wheat Ridge, CO: Author.

About the Midwest Nursing Research Society

The Midwest Nursing Research Society (MNRS) is a nursing research organization with a broad membership of nurses, nurse scientists, and students, others from the United States and beyond.

MNRS Mission:
- The mission of MNRS is to advance science, transform practice, and enhance careers through a network of scholars.

MNRS Vision:
- The premiere society that develops scholars, drives science, and leads innovation to improve the health of all people.

Membership in MNRS provides valuable benefits:
- Subscription to the Western Journal of Nursing Research, the official journal of MNRS
- Invitation to submit abstracts for symposia, papers or poster presentations at the Annual MNRS Conference
- Opportunity to join research interest groups and interact with colleagues with similar interests
- Membership directory listing
- Opportunity to submit proposals for dissertation and seed grants
- Awards program that recognized nurse researchers at several points in their careers including students and senior scientists
- Discounted registration fees for the Annual conference and Pre-conferences
- Thriving emerging scholars network for students and early career nurse researchers
- Opportunities to develop leadership skills

NOTES

Made in the USA
San Bernardino, CA
17 July 2020